NATURE'S NUTRIENT

Understanding The Vital Role of Fruits and Vegetables

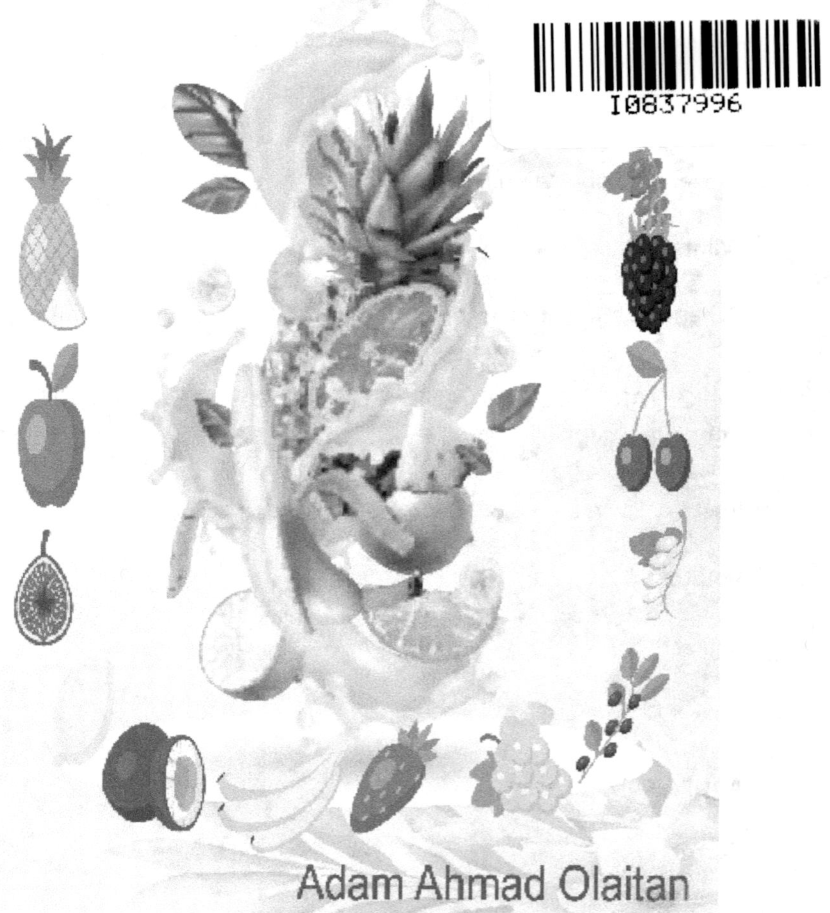

Adam Ahmad Olaitan

TABLE OF CONTENTS

About the book

This book "***Nature's Nutrients: Understanding the vital role of fruits and vegetables***" offers a comprehensive exploration of fruits and vegetables as vital components of human nutrition. It delves into the definitions, composition, and the scientific importance of these natural foods in addressing health deficiencies. By breaking down the essential nutrients—such as vitamins, minerals, fiber, and antioxidants—found in various fruits and vegetables, the book explains their critical role in maintaining overall health.

Through an informative discussion of how these nutrients support bodily functions, the book highlights the direct link between a balanced intake of fruits and vegetables and the prevention of nutrient deficiencies. Topics covered include the specific benefits of different fruits and vegetables, their nutritional profiles, and the overall importance of incorporating them into daily diets

Perfect for nutrition enthusiasts and anyone interested in improving their health, this book offers a solid understanding of how fruits and vegetables can help promote wellness and prevent deficiency-related health issues.

Why Fruit and Vegetables

Take into consideration the likely aspects of your current diet and way of life. Lift your hand on the chance that any of these focuses concern you:

You are in a state of chronic stress due to work, family, and financial pressures.

You spend more than eight hours a day looking at a computer screen, with a hunched back, staring at a bright screen.

You spend barely any time outside.

You drink contaminated tap water.

You breathe harmful smog-filled air.

You are constantly stressed, don't get enough sleep, overindulge in sugary foods, and don't eat enough greens.

You then wonder why we aren't feeling 100%!

Even if you were correct about the majority of these points, the reality is that our contemporary lifestyles are absolutely terrible for our health.

This is true right down to the fact that most of us are just too comfortable. Our bodies have forgotten how to deal with stress and difficulty because we have "adapted" to a comfortable, domesticated lifestyle.

Take, for instance, going outside. Because most of us don't do this enough, we don't get enough of the important stimulus of sunlight. This helps the body make vitamin D, which controls things like hormone production, sleep, mood, and even appetite!

Our body loses some of its natural rhythm and certain processes are disrupted without that crucial input, which is referred to in the scientific literature as an "external zeitgebers."

But there's also the huge advantage of being outside in the cold. Being outside boosts testosterone levels, strengthens our immune system, and even improves our ability to regulate our own body temperature even when the sun isn't out.

Given that we never exercise this aspect of our health, is it any wonder that we always feel "stuffy"?

In any event, investing energy barefooted on the earth (which trains minuscule muscles in the foot), in any event, plunging into water and pausing our breathing (which prepares our lungs and further develops our CO2 balance) these are everything our bodies ache for. We are not providing that, either. As a result, our bodies are significantly deteriorating.

Indeed, it's all excellent and well me letting you know that you ought to be sorting out over the course of the day, that you ought to eat impeccably, and that you ought to be taking long swims in freezing cold water in the first part of the day. Issue is, we lack the capacity to deal with that and our bodies are presently maladapted to the point that they wouldn't deal with it.

In any event, fixing your eating routine - disposing of all that undesirable handled food, lessening the quantity of complete calories, getting more fiber, decreasing basic carbs… it's a lot of work and can get very convoluted. Which is the reason the best spot to begin is by fixing one of the greatest issues with current life. That is: the absence of micronutrient.

Micronutrient are nutrients, minerals, amino acids, unsaturated fats, cell reinforcements, and other dynamic fixings in our food that our body utilizes for a wide range of purposes.

What many individuals don't understand is that we in a real sense are what we eat. You hear this a ton, yet many individuals expect that it is a sort of similitude. However, no: your body takes in the supplements that you consume and afterward it utilizes those supplements to modify your body as a matter of fact.

For instance, your bones are made mostly from calcium, and magnesium. These likewise help to reinforce your connective tissue (ligaments and tendons), your teeth, and your nails. Connective tissues likewise benefit from any semblance of collagen (found in bone stock) which additionally assists with working on your skin.

If by some stroke of good luck, you could get more products of the soil in your eating regimen then, at that point, you would turn into the best and best adaptation of yourself. Also, that thus could then give you the energy and determination to wrap up.

Foods grown from the ground could supercharge your digestion, assisting you with consuming significantly more fat!

As we will find in the remainder of this book, fixing your admission of products of the soil needn't bother with being troublesome. In the event that you are vital, simplifying only a couple of changes can change your wellbeing and prosperity.

This book will likewise frame a significant number of the other astounding and complex manners by which organic products can work on your wellbeing and execution - some of which are totally extraordinary to the manner in which you look and feel.

You'll know exactly which foods grown from the ground that can fix any of your

Current illnesses, and you'll know definitively how to get them. How about we get to it.

Composition of Fruits and Vegetables

Fruits and vegetables contain many vitamins and minerals that are good for your health. Many of these are antioxidants, and may reduce the risk of many diseases: -

Vitamin A (beta-carotene)

Vitamin C

Vitamin E

Magnesium

Zinc

Phosphorous

Folic acid

It is with doubt that fruit and vegetables contain useful ingredients needed for your well being

Let's take a closer look at the specific advantages of fruits and vegetables before proceeding any further. Furthermore, obviously, the primary spot to begin is by taking a gander at the nutrient substance.

You might be surprised to learn that vitamins were first discovered less than a century ago. Until they were formally found, specialists realized that specific food sources assisted with specific states of being, however they didn't have the foggiest idea why.

For instance, in 1975, the British Navy began carrying a supply of limes because doctors had discovered that sailors who consumed the juice or ate a certain amount each day avoided developing scurvy.

However, the term "vitamins," which later became known as vitamins, was not coined until 1912 by

Casimir Funk, who was working in the United Kingdom and later in the United States.

Since then, research on vitamins has progressed, and while most of us are familiar with the names of the most common vitamins, we may not always know what they do. Vitamins come in two varieties. Vitamins that dissolve in water and fat are the two types.

Fat Soluble Vitamins

Vitamins A, D, E, and K are the most well-known fat-soluble vitamins.

Vitamin A keeps the skin moist and maintains the suppleness, smoothness, and suppleness of the mucus membranes. In addition, it helps keep the reproductive system in good health and encourages healthy bone growth in low light. Whole milk, butter, eggs, and liver are all good sources of vitamin A. Carotenoids, which are red, yellow, and dark green fruits and vegetables, are a type of vitamin A.

The absorption of calcium by the body requires vitamin D. As a result, it shares the same role as calcium in maintaining healthy bones and teeth. However, both are required and beneficial. "Fortified" foods like cereals and fat spreads frequently contain vitamin D. Because sunlight is the primary source of vitamin D, it is also referred to as the "sunshine vitamin."

The nervous system, reproductive system, and muscle health are all aided by vitamin E. It also fights free radicals. Because it is fat-soluble, it is stored in the body and can help shield cells from free radicals, which can harm other cells. Whole grains, nuts, wheat germ oil, and green leafy vegetables are all good sources of vitamin E.

Blood clotting is mainly caused by vitamin K. If you didn't have it, you would risk dying every time you cut yourself. Additionally, kidney tissues and bone are made by this vitamin. Fruit, cheese, cereals, dark green leafy vegetables, and liver are all good sources of vitamin K. Additionally, it is produced by friendly bacteria in the intestines.

The obvious advantage of fat-soluble vitamins is that if your diet is temporarily lacking in one of these vitamins, you are less likely to suffer a deficiency. The disadvantage of these types of vitamins is that if you consume too much of one of them, then your body is unable to flush out the surplus and you could suffer from a vitamin overdose.

Water Soluble Vitamins

Vitamin C and all of the B vitamins are the most well-known water-soluble vitamins.

Ascorbic acid is another name for vitamin C. It helps to maintain the muscle, fat, and bone framework, or connective tissues, in the body. It likewise assists with recuperating wounds by accelerating the development of new cells, is an enemy of oxidant, and assists the body with engrossing iron. Vitamin C also helps the body fight infections by protecting the body's immune system. Fruit, juices from fruits, and vegetables are all good sources of vitamin C.

B1 (thiamin), B2 (riboflavin), B3 (niacin), B6 (pyridoxine), and B12 (cyanocobalamin) are members of the B vitamin family. The primary objective of this class of vitamins is to ensure proper body function.

The body needs vitamin B1 to break down fats, alcohol, and carbohydrates into energy. Lean pork, unrefined cereals, seeds, and nuts all contain this vitamin.

B2 helps the body use and digest proteins, carbohydrates, and fats, and regulates appetite. Fish, poultry, meat, milk, and eggs all contain B2. This vitamin can be found in abundance in dark leafy vegetables and in brewer's yeast.

B3 is necessary for healthy growth and the passage of oxygen through the body's tissues. Additionally, it is accountable for sustaining a healthy appetite. Meat, cereals with vitamin B3 added, and fortified bread are all good sources.

B6 is responsible for obtaining energy and nutrients from food. It forestalls coronary illness by eliminating overabundance homocysteine from the blood. Soy beans, nuts, eggs, whole grains, lamb, port, chicken, fish, and milk are all sources of B6.

B12 aids in the production of healthy red blood cells. Additionally, it enables the body to transmit messages among its nerve cells, making it possible for us to hear, move, think, and carry out the usual activities of daily life. It is produced by bacteria in the small intestine of the body. Although this vitamin is water-soluble, it can be stored in the liver and is added to many foods, including cereals. Eggs, milk, poultry, fish, and milk are all sources of B12.

The disadvantage of these vitamins is that you may need to take in larger amounts as it cannot be stored. If your diet is deficient in one of these vitamins, even for a short time, you may suffer symptoms of vitamin deficiency as a result, there is no back up supply stored in your body.

Although both fruits and vegetables are full of both vitamins and minerals, fruits typically have a higher concentration of vitamins than vegetables.

Therefore, a good starting question might be: What is the distinction between a mineral and a vitamin?

Though nutrients are natural and subsequently are ordinarily very unpredictable (they can be separated by any semblance of intensity, air, and corrosive), minerals are on the other hand inorganic. In point of fact, a mineral can actually be a metal or a rock, which you would never really consider to be a fundamental component of who you are.

Minerals, on the other hand, are necessary for the human body to function properly. For example, the body uses iron, a crucial mineral, to make hemoglobin, which is the oxygen-carrying red blood cells that travel throughout the body.

It would be impossible to provide energy throughout the body for the numerous essential functions that take place, such as breathing and digestion.

Minerals typically play a slightly more fundamental role in the body's structural components, particularly the harder ones. Minerals, for instance, are what make up bones, tendons, and ligaments.

Minerals, on the other hand, also play a role in conduction. After all, the body is powered by electricity, and maintaining the appropriate charge is essential to the healthy operation of our brain and muscles.

Because the body cannot correctly communicate with the muscles, an imbalance in sodium and potassium can lead to cramping. Similarly, an absence of calcium can diminish strength as taking care of the charge in the muscle cells is required

Other Essential Micronutrient

Fruits and vegetables not only contain a lot of vitamins and minerals, but they also contain a lot of the two other important nutrients. Other important nutrients include: the essential amino acids and fatty acids

Amino acids are, in essence, the components that make up proteins. Many of these are found in meat, which our bodies then use to rebuild tissue by breaking down the components. We were shown at the beginning of this book that we are literally what we eat!

Amino acids, and by extension proteins, are crucial for athletes and bodybuilders attempting to build muscle. According to research, athletes should consume 1 gram of protein for every 1 pound of body weight. Additionally, protein has a thermogenic effect, which means that simply digesting it will actually result in the burning of calories. Protein is also much more difficult to convert into fat, for instance.

Consequently, many individuals will be working diligently attempting to find wellsprings of protein from meat and will eat a lot of chicken to fabricate greater muscles. This could become a lot of work! However, despite the fact that fruits are slightly superior in this regard, they neglect the fact that vegetables and even fruits contain protein.

Think about how much protein is in the broccoli on the chicken's side, not just the protein from the protein shakes and chicken.

Amino acids likewise play a large group of different jobs in the body and are utilized to deliver stomach related proteins, synapses (mind synthetic compounds) and considerably more. They can also create, for example.

Lastly, vegetables and fruits are rich in essential fatty acids. These essential fats aid in the absorption of other fruits and vegetables and provide a variety of additional benefits, including improving brain function (the brain is made of a lot of fat!).

Omega 3 is one of the most potent essential fatty acids available and offers a plethora of incredible advantages. Omega 3 is often thought to be found in fish, but it can also be found in high amounts in

seaweed, hemp seeds, walnuts, kidney beans,
soybeans, and other foods.

Importance of Fruit and Vegetables for Good Athletic Performance

When you think of a diet for muscle building, you probably think of the usual choices. It is likely that you will concentrate primarily on protein sources like eggs, tuna, and chicken. Meta and steamed rice should be the only foods an athlete eats, right?

However, this is far from the only kind of food that can help you build muscle and perform better. In fact, if you want to compete in bodybuilding, sprinting, swimming, long-distance running, or any other kind of athletic activity, you need to eat a well-balanced diet that includes a wide variety of food groups. Specifically, it is essential you get your leafy foods.

Are you interested in enhancing your athletic performance with supplements? You might find it interesting to learn that eating fruits and vegetables can actually be more effective, cost much less, and have a plethora of other amazing benefits for your health!

Here are some illustrations.

Beets

Beets are without a doubt one of the most essential vegetables for athletes of all kinds and for building muscle.

This is due to the fact that beets are one of the foods that raise nitric oxide the most effectively in the world. Nitric oxide is a "vasodilator" by nature. This indicates that it may have the potential to widen or dilate the blood vessels (arteries and veins), thereby facilitating the circulation of oxygen and nutrients throughout the body.

As a result, the muscles receive more nutrients and oxygen for improved recovery during training. You might be able to lift for more reps, run longer distances, and recover faster as a result of this.

Potato

Carbohydrates are frequently portrayed as undesirables, despite their crucial role in muscle development and physical training as a whole. Potatoes are a good source of carbohydrates due to their high fiber content, high vitamin C content (which aids in recovery), and low-calorie content. Consume after an exercise and the energy will go directly to the muscles as opposed to the midsection.

Spinach

Spinach is a high-protein vegetable that is also a good source of phytoecdysteroids. Although these do not share any similarities with anabolic steroids, some studies suggest that they are a good option for encouraging the production of testosterone and muscle mass.

Kale

Kale has the most calcium of any vegetable. Calcium is actually very important for your workouts because it not only helps to strengthen your bones but also strengthens your connective tissue. It also helps to strengthen contractions, which means you can work out with more explosive power.

Because it is low in calories and high in protein, kale is very popular right now. However, a disgrace it costs a fair piece!

Mushrooms

Although they are not technically vegetables or fruits, mushrooms can be found in the same aisle and are safe for vegans, so they should be included. In addition to being an excellent protein source, mushrooms offer a plethora of additional health advantages. They have a lot of minerals in them, they can help you recover from training, and a lot more!

It's only a matter of time before health food stores start selling mushroom protein shakes!

The other astounding advantage of mushrooms is that they contain vitamin D.

They're one of a handful of the dietary wellsprings of vitamin D! (One more is oily fish).

This is significant because vitamin D is regarded as a master hormone regulator and is specifically responsible for encouraging the production of testosterone, one of the most important anabolic hormones for muscle building and fat burning.

Carrots

Carrots are generally good for you and a good source of vitamin A, C, and K. But the lutein in them is really exciting because it may help you get more energy and make your mitochondria work better!

Your cells' energy factories are your mitochondria, which convert glucose into ATP (ATP is your body's usable form of energy and glucose is the sugar from carbohydrates). This means that carrots and other sources of lutein can actually help you run faster and burn more calories even when you're not working out!

In one study, rats were given lutein, which can only be absorbed by eating fat, like milk, and it was found that they started running long distances in their wheel on their own, burning a lot more fat in the process.

Apples

It contains a lot of vitamin C, which is another important vitamin for strengthening the immune system and assisting athletes in training for longer periods of time and harder.

In addition, when combined with zinc, vitamin C boosts the production of testosterone and nitric oxide as well as increases serotonin, which aids in mental recovery.

Apples also contain a lot of fiber, which can help lower blood pressure and improve bowel movements as well as food absorption. Additionally, fiber is essential for maintaining a healthy microbiome, which in turn can promote a strong immune system, improved mood, weight loss, and many other benefits.

Fruit and Vegetables - An Improvement to Beauty, Energy and Mood

So, you're not particularly interested in weight loss? Perhaps you are already happy with the size you are? (Good for you!)

Maybe you're not an athlete? Maybe you don't have noticeable health problems?

Look, fruit and vegetables are for everyone. And just to ram that point home, here are some more examples of fruit and vegetables with wildly varying different healthy benefits

Strawberry Create Energy

As a study in the Journal of Agricultural and Food Chemistry notes, strawberries are a good source of minerals, vitamin C, and folates. They also contain phenols, which are essential antioxidants that may help the body create energy at the cellular level.

People can add strawberries to many dishes, and a handful may also be an easy snack to add to a diet.

Oranges For Mood Swing

Most people enjoy oranges for their taste, which comes from the antioxidant vitamin C. Vitamin C may help reduce oxidative stress in the body and prevent fatigue.

A study in the journal Antioxidants notes that young adult male students who have higher levels of vitamin C may also have a better mood and may be less likely to experience confusion, anger, or depression.

Berries are Sweet but Less Sugary

Berries, including blueberries, raspberries, and blackberries, may be a good energy boosting food when the body is craving something sweet.

Dark berries tend to be higher in natural antioxidants than lighter-colored ones, which may reduce inflammation and fatigue in the body. They also tend to have less sugar than sweeter fruits, while still satisfying a craving for a sweet taste.

Fruit and vegetables can assist with making you look more lovely. What's more, that is genuine even of something as straightforward as your unassuming broccoli!

Broccoli is maybe somewhat less 'colorful' when contrasted with a portion of the other superfood products of the soil on this rundown. However, don't let that fool you: this is as yet an unbelievably nutritious food that everybody ought to get a greater amount of.

Yet again first off, broccoli is a decent wellspring of fiber and can assist with working on your processing, your defecations, and substantially more. In addition, however, broccoli is likewise exceptionally high in vitamin K, ascorbic acid, fiber, potassium, collagen, iron, calcium, and then some.

How about we start by plunging into that collagen. This is the kind of thing that we all need yet not very many of us get. Collagen has been displayed to further develop cerebrum capability and battle against

Alzheimer's, it additionally assists with lessening back torment, further develops skin versatility, fortifies the nails, battles cracked stomach condition, battles knee torment, and for the most part strengthens your ligaments, tendons, and bones.

To this end feasts, for example, bone stock was amazingly great for us. Furthermore, presently late exploration is proposing a much more impressive explanation that collagen may be so significant.

Pregnant moms ought to investigate eating more broccoli. That is on the grounds that both broccoli and numerous plates of mixed greens leaves are a decent wellspring of folate, which is something that all moms are prescribed to eat.

Not getting sufficient folate expands the gamble of confusions in pregnancy, and that is the reason a ton of moms will attempt to get all the more misleadingly using pregnancy supplements.

This is where it means quite a bit to bring up the huge benefits of getting a greater number of supplements from your eating regimen as opposed to from supplements. While it is actually the case that you can profit from supplements, these are planned to enhance your standard eating regimen.

In other words that they ought to be taken notwithstanding your customary eating regimen, as opposed to as another option. Supplements from your eating regimen are undeniably more compelling than those taken in pill structure, as they are joined with various different supplements, fats, strands, and different components.

Together, this assistance to further develop assimilation of the critical components and that makes them considerably more compelling. What is perceived is that the human body developed while being presented to these food sources and thus is ideally intended to remove the healthy benefit here.

Consuming supplements in an engineered form isn't planned. This is the reason so many tell you not to take nutrient tablets while starving'. They simply work better as food varieties

Cayenne pepper meanwhile is another great tool in the battle against inflammation. This is a compound that makes food spicy and is widely found in ointments and creams due to its anti-inflammation effects. It's a common pain- relief too as it depletes nerve cells of the chemical 'substance P'. Substance P causes both inflammation and the sensation of pain, so this is a great thing to add to your diet if you do suffer from a condition like fibromyalgia or arthritis.

Cayenne also comes packed with flavonoids and carotenoids. These are antioxidants that prevent cellular damage, thereby further combating against inflammation.

Cayenne pepper also has a number of other impressive benefits. It has been shown to be an effective appetite suppressant for instance, meaning that if you are someone who struggles to stick to a diet, you might start finding it a little easier to be disciplined and thereby hopefully see the weight begin to fall off.

At the same time, cayenne pepper may help to improve digestion. This is important because better digestion doesn't only give you more energy and prevent discomfort, but it also helps you to better absorb nutrients from your food. That means that all the benefits you're getting from the other superfoods on this list will then be turned up to 11.

What's more is that cayenne pepper has also been shown to increase testosterone. This of course is the hormone that most of us know as the 'male hormone' and is responsible for the male sex drive, as well as many of the differences between men and women. Increasing testosterone in men increases muscle tone, reduces fat storage, raises aggression, aids with recovery, fortifies the immune system and more. Men who don't get enough testosterone will exhibit signs of depression, low energy, low mood, and low sex drive. They also struggle with weight gain and low muscle mass. Conversely, men with high testosterone exhibit the traits that we associate with the classic 'alpha male' along with toned and powerful physiques.   This is why so many men try to augment their natural testosterone production through the use of steroids and other drugs – despite those carrying numerous health warnings and serious dangers.   The really worrying part is that testosterone in men is increasing across the globe by 1% a year. This is partly due to the use of feminine products and their impact on our water, along with a host of other problems (certain plastics and our generally inactive lifestyles). But diet plays a BIG part in it too. Time to start eating a little less processed food, and a little more cayenne.

Fruit and Vegetables Can Successfully Improve Your Health

At this point, you should have a comprehensive idea of the best reasons to ensure you are getting enough fruits and vegetables in your diet. These can enhance your health in a myriad way, and if you are currently feeling tired, moody, unwell, or even depressed, it's highly likely that you have a deficiency in at least one of these micronutrients. And this should come as no surprise – given that the vast majority of people do have some kind of deficiency these days.

The next question is how you should be gently integrating these fruits and vegetables. Are there any drawbacks? How many do you need precisely? Can you just use a vitamin tablet instead?

How is it done?

The Point is Assortment rather than searching out individual various leafy foods, what is far ideal is to just expect to get the greatest assortment you can in your eating regimen. By doing this, you will cover the biggest range of fixings, and consequently get the biggest scope of various advantages from your eating regimen.

You could find the best superfood vegetable on the planet, yet in the event that that was all you ate then you wouldn't get all that much advantage - in light of the fact that you'd just be getting a lot of those equivalent fixings.

We don't consider food varieties, for example, apples as being super food sources, but since they contain a lot of L-ascorbic acid (cell reinforcement, helps testosterone, supports nitric oxide development, produces serotonin), epicatechin, they are similarly essentially as noteworthy as those more colorful thoughts.

In addition, in the event that you eat three unique products of the soil, the scope of supplements you get will be far more prominent.

Concentrates on show too, that our microbiome - the solid microorganisms living in our guts - benefit in particular from a shifted diet. The more noteworthy the scope of food varieties you eat, the more grounded your stomach wellbeing will be - bringing about weight reduction, more energy, better temperament, and that's only the tip of the iceberg.

At long last, by planning to simply "eat loads of products of the soil" you can lessen how much thought this diet support includes, which thus will assist you with being bound to adhere to your new responsibility.

Don't overdo it

That said, you can do yourself damage by consuming too many fruits and vegetables. Or to be a little more specific, it is relatively easy to cause harm by consuming too much fruit.

That's because fruit is highly acidic and packed with sugar. Both these things make it damaging to your teeth in particular. Many people who switch to diets that are primarily focused on the use of smoothies will end up developing serious tooth problems!

One solution to this is to avoid drinking too much fruit juice or too many fruit smoothies. Instead, focus on drinking vegetable smoothies, which typically contain a lot less sugar.

Another consideration is that fruits and vegetables are still a source of calories. This is especially true for things like avocados, which have become all the rage recently. While avocados are great for boosting testosterone (thanks to their healthy saturated fat content), and while they are useful for those trying to avoid carbs, they can still make you fat!

Don't make the mistake of thinking that "fruits and vegetables are healthy and therefore can't make you fat."

The truth is that they still contain calories and you still need to track and manage those calories to avoid unwanted weight.

Live Longer with Antioxidants

Antioxidants are found naturally in our diet and are also a key feature of many supplements. Antioxidants are something of a buzz word these days and antioxidant vitamins and minerals as well as a range of Naka Herb supplements are highly popular.

What is the reason for this? And what precisely are antioxidants? Here we will look a little at how a cell works, how a cell dies and why antioxidants are so important.

Our cells are made up of various parts but all you need to know about in this instance is the cell wall and the nucleus. The cell wall, surrounded by mitochondria, is the part of the cell that of course holds everything together and gives the cell its round appearance.

Meanwhile the nucleus is the center of the cell, which is often referred to as the 'control center'. Here is where the DNA is stored, the 'blueprint' that tells the cell what it looks like, how to behave and where the other important cells go in the body.

Unfortunately, though, what's also in our body is 'free radicals' and this is where the antioxidant vitamins and minerals and the Naka Herb supplements come in. Essentially free radicals are substances that travel around the body and damage the cells. They are a by-product of many things from simply breathing (oxygen is reactive and damages cells) to getting too much direct sunlight (the UV waves in the sunlight are radioactive and can damage our cell walls too).

These free radicals then do a lot of serious damage in the body and are enough to eventually make our skin look older – because the damage though microscopic can eventually add up to be visible to the naked eye and this goes for skin cells as well. This is why lots of exposure to the sun will make you look good and tanned in the short term, but ultimately result in your skin appearing wrinkled and leathery.

More seriously though, eventually these free radicals will break all the way through the cell walls, and this will mean that they reach the nucleus where the DNA is housed. If they reach this then they can cause damage to your actual genetic code and this results in mutation which changes the expression of the cell and renders it unable to do its job.

Because cells reproduce by splitting (mitosis) this then means that when the cell splits it will copy the DNA across and you will have two fault cells. Your immune system tries to stop this and can be aided if you buy herbs online, but it would be better of course if it could be prevented. Because those dead cells as they spread become cancer, and can eventually lead to the failure of whole organs.

Antioxidant vitamins and minerals from fruits, vegetables, and even supplements will help you to do this – by destroying the free radicals on impact thereby preventing them ever causing that damage. These will then slow your visible aging and help to deter cancer – not bad!

The Strategy to Balanced Diet

So how would you build the assortment? Here are a few simple tips that will assist you with doing that without adding a ton of stress to your next shopping trip:

Make loads of stews, hot pots, and Italian dishes. On the off chance that you're cooking something like a bolognaise, it's entirely simple to toss a lot of foods grown from the ground into a pot with some mince.

To make this much simpler, take a stab at grinding things like carrot (so you needn't bother with striping), and utilize frozen fixings like mushrooms, peas, and sweetcorn.

Make bunches of plates of mixed greens! A simple method for making a virus lunch is to get some serving of mixed greens leaves, toss on a few yams, cut some cucumber, and add a spot of lemon. This can go on almost ANYTHING you cook. Pick child leaf spinach and you'll get iron and folate. Then fluctuate which leaf you utilize like clockwork.

Hold up! While doing this, concoct huge clumps of food sources and afterward freeze them in heaps of separately partitioned Tupperware. Then all you want to do is to thaw out every one as you come to eat it.

Make smoothies! These are very simple to deliver - toss a lot of foods grown from the ground/vegetables in and hit mix. They likewise give a gigantic increase in astonishing advantages. The absolute most fiery and blissful individuals I know consume day to day smoothies!

Purchase products of the soil out. A ton of bistros sell organic products at the counter, and the equivalent is valid in numerous merchants. Rather than purchasing a chocolate nibble, simply purchase the most intriguing looking organic product you can find!

Multivitamins Supplement

A multivitamin supplement is an enhancement that contains an equilibrium of various supplements. You could normally see one that contains a mix of L-ascorbic acid, D, A, and B complex. In like manner, multi mineral enhancements could contain Iron, Magnesium, Potassium, Calcium, and Zinc for "sound bones and chemical equilibrium."

Are these items comparably great as the "genuine article?"

Indeed, and negative.

From one perspective, you can assimilate and profit from supplements. Certain individuals will let you know that this isn't accurate, however there are a few valid justifications to accept in any case. As far as one might be concerned, did you have any idea that there really exist a few items that are intended to supplant your whole eating routine? These incorporate any semblance of Soylent, which apparently contains each and every supplement the body needs, all decent impeccably.

Is it a smart thought? Not in any way shape or form! Yet, what to zero in on right presently is that individuals who utilize this item make due… and they're very sound! What's more, in light of that, we can along these lines state without a doubt that multivitamins can likewise be retained.

In any case, there's a trick. The first of these gets is that a multivitamin is simply going to be essentially as great as the individual who planned it. We saw with lutein and other fat-solvent nutrients for instance. These need a wellspring of fat to be ingested into the circulation system. Get them from regular food sources, and odds are good that the wellspring of fat will be incorporated. Get them from a nutrient enhancement and they could not.

Comparative cooperation likewise exists between numerous different nutrients and minerals, where one will help the other to effectively be ingested more. Similarly, various nutrients and minerals ingest at various rates, thus in a perfect world ought not be joined into a solitary item.

Then there are different things that products of the soil contain that do us great - like fiber, amino acids, and that's only the tip of the iceberg. Furthermore, there's the little reality that all foods grown from the ground contain substances that we don't completely have any idea or maybe aren't even mindful of.

We just barely found the phenomenal advantages of lutein (that go past eye wellbeing). So, eating genuine foods grown from the ground is Consistently best.

However, in the event that the decision comes down to utilizing an enhancement or not getting those valuable supplements by any means… then the enhancement is obviously better. As a matter of fact, an enhancement can be an exceptionally helpful and simple method for getting what you want in your eating regimen, or can be thought of as a "back up."

Closing Reflection

This book has highlighted the incredible power of fruits and vegetables in combating health deficiencies and improving overall well-being. These natural foods, abundant in essential nutrients such as vitamins, minerals, antioxidants, and fiber, are indispensable for maintaining good health. Through a deeper understanding of their composition and importance, we can appreciate how these nutrient-packed plants provide the body with the tools it needs to function optimally, prevent disease, and promote longevity.

We've explored how specific fruits and vegetables target common health issues like anemia, vitamin deficiencies, and digestive problems, while also supporting vital systems such as cardiovascular health, immune function, and brain health. The diversity of nutrients present in different fruits and vegetables not only addresses immediate health concerns but also works synergistically to boost overall vitality, energy levels, and long-term wellness.

Moreover, adopting a diet rich in fruits and vegetables goes beyond personal health. It contributes to a more sustainable and environmentally friendly lifestyle. By choosing whole, plant-based foods, we reduce our dependence on processed and nutrient-depleted foods that have contributed to many modern health challenges. With every meal, you have the opportunity to make a positive impact not just on your body, but on the world around you.

The key takeaway is that a diet abundant in fruits and vegetables is more than just a solution to deficiencies—it is a lifelong investment in health. The vibrant colors, flavors, and textures of these foods are nature's way of delivering a variety of nutrients in their most accessible and enjoyable forms. From leafy greens to citrus fruits, root vegetables to berries, every serving nourishes and rejuvenates the body.

As you move forward from here, consider how you can integrate these nutrient-dense foods more intentionally into your daily life. Experiment with new recipes, explore seasonal produce, and diversify your plate to ensure that your body receives a broad spectrum of nutrients. In doing so, you will not only prevent health deficiencies but also cultivate a lifestyle that promotes long-term vitality and well-being.

Remember, the journey to optimal health starts with small, sustainable steps. Let the knowledge and insights from this book empower you to make fruits and vegetables the cornerstone of your diet, unlocking their full potential to support and enhance your health for years to come.

About the Author

Adam Ahmad Olaitan is a passionate advocate for holistic health and nutrition, with a deep focus on the vital role that fruits and vegetables play in human wellness. He has spent years researching and educating others on the importance of natural foods in preventing nutrient deficiencies and promoting overall health.

Driven by a belief in the healing power of nature, he has written extensively on how plant-based nutrition can be an accessible and sustainable solution to modern health challenges. Through his work, he aims to inspire individuals to embrace healthier lifestyles by incorporating more nutrient-dense, natural foods into their diets.

When not writing or researching, ***Ahmad*** enjoys activities related to food, wellness, or nature, further deepening his connection to the natural world. This book is a culmination of years of dedication to health education, offering readers a well-researched guide to improving their well-being through fruits and vegetables.